44 Testicular Cancer Juice Recipes:

Naturally Prevent and Treat Testicular Cancer without Recurring to Medical Treatments or Pills

By

Joe Correa CSN

COPYRIGHT

This publication is designed to provide accurate and authoritative information in regard to the subject matter covered. It is sold with the understanding that neither the author nor the publisher is engaged in rendering medical advice. If medical advice or assistance is needed, consult with a doctor. This book is considered a guide and should not be used in any way detrimental to your health. Consult with a physician before starting this nutritional plan to make sure it's right for you.

ACKNOWLEDGEMENTS

This book is dedicated to my friends and family that have had mild or serious illnesses so that you may find a solution and make the necessary changes in your life.

44 Testicular Cancer Juice Recipes:

Naturally Prevent and Treat Testicular Cancer without Recurring to Medical Treatments or Pills

By

Joe Correa CSN

CONTENTS

ABOUT THE AUTHOR

After years of Research, I honestly believe in the positive effects that proper nutrition can have over the body and mind. My knowledge and experience has helped me live healthier throughout the years and which I have shared with family and friends. The more you know about eating and drinking healthier, the sooner you will want to change your life and eating habits.

Nutrition is a key part in the process of being healthy and living longer so get started today. The first step is the most important and the most significant.

INTRODUCTION

44 Testicular Cancer Juice Recipes: Naturally Prevent and Treat Testicular Cancer without Recurring to Medical Treatments or Pills

By Joe Correa CSN

The testicular cancer is the most common cancer in the male reproductive system. It is usually detected by a person discovering some form of abnormality in their testicles.

This disease starts with an abnormal cell growth in one or both testicles. Compared to other cancers, this abnormality is relatively rare. In the US, this type of cancer is most common in males between the ages of 15-45. Fortunately, testicular cancer can be effectively treated with a 95% average survival rate. Just like every other cancer, this type of cancer is usually treated with radiation therapy, chemotherapy, and surgery.

There are some risk factors that increase your chances of getting testicular cancer. If you fall into any of these categories, you should definitely pay These risk factors include:

- **Age.** Testicular cancer is most common in men between 15-45 years. This, however, doesn't mean that older men shouldn't visit a doctor if they detect something suspicious.
- **Undescended testicle.** This is a condition where one or both testicles didn't move down into the scrotum. It is highly related to testicular cancer and you should keep that in mind if you fall into this category.
- **Family history.** Just like most types of cancer, if you have a family history of this disease, you're more likely to get testicular cancer.
- **HIV.** People who suffer from HIV have a high risk of developing a testicular cancer.
  I have to point out that even if you don't fall into any of these categories, it doesn't mean you shouldn't do whatever you can to prevent cancer.

Your diet, lifestyle, and overall health condition are extremely important in order to prevent testicular cancer. There are certain foods that are proven to be extremely effective against this type of cancer. These foods include basil, garlic, onions, chives, berries of all kinds, green and black tea, apples, turmeric, cumin, broccoli, cabbage, Brussels sprouts, cauliflower, citrus fruits, etc.

Having this in mind, I have created this cookbook with delicious juices recipes that will help you heal your body and prevent having cancer. Within just a couple of minutes, you will have a truly valuable nutritional drink that will boost your immune system and give your body everything it needs in order to function properly.

44 TESTICULAR CANCER JUICE RECIPES: NATURALLY PREVENT AND TREAT TESTICULAR CANCER WITHOUT RECURRING TO MEDICAL TREATMENTS OR PILLS

1.   Blueberry Basil Juice

Ingredients:

1 cup of blueberries

1 cup of fresh basil, torn

1 cup of strawberries, sliced

1 whole lemon, peeled

1 small Granny Smith's apple, cored

Preparation:

Place the blueberries in a colander and rinse under cold running water. Slightly drain and set aside.

Wash the basil thoroughly and torn with hands. Set aside.

Wash the strawberries and remove the stems. Cut into slices and fill the measuring cup. Reserve the rest for later.

Peel the lemon and cut lengthwise in half. Set aside.

Wash the apple and cut in half. Remove the core and cut into bite-sized pieces. Set aside.

Now, combine blueberries, basil, strawberries, lemon, and apple in a juicer and process until juiced. Transfer to a serving glass and add few ice cubes.

Serve immediately.

Nutritional information per serving: Kcal: 193, Protein: 4.3g, Carbs: 60.1g, Fats: 1.6g

2.   Tomato Mustard Green Juice

Ingredients:

1 medium-sized Roma tomato, chopped

1 cup of mustard greens, torn

1 cup of fresh spinach, torn

1 large carrot, sliced

1 tsp of fresh rosemary, finely chopped

Preparation:

Wash the tomato and place it in a bowl. Cut into bite-sized pieces and make sure to reserve tomato juices while cutting. Set aside.

Wash mustard greens and spinach thoroughly under cold running water. Slightly drain and torn with hands. Set aside.

Wash and peel the carrot. Cut into thin slices and set aside.

Now, combine tomato, mustard greens, spinach, carrot, and rosemary in a juicer and process until juiced. Transfer to a serving glass and stir in the reserved tomato juice. Refrigerate for 15 minutes before serving.

Enjoy!

Nutritional information per serving: Kcal: 74, Protein: 9.4g, Carbs: 21.9g, Fats: 1.5g

3.   Watercress Celery Juice

Ingredients:

2 cups of fresh watercress, chopped

2 large celery stalks, chopped

1 cup of cucumber, sliced

1 whole lime, peeled

¼ tsp of turmeric, ground

1 oz of water

Preparation:

Place the watercress in a large colander. Rinse under cold running water. Torn with hands and set aside.

Wash the celery stalks and cut into bite-sized pieces. Set aside.

Wash the cucumber and cut into thin slices. Fill the measuring cup and reserve the rest for later.

Peel the lime and cut lengthwise in half. Set aside.

Now, combine watercress, celery, cucumber, and lime in a juicer. Process until juiced. Transfer to a serving glass and stir in the turmeric and water.

Refrigerate for 10 minutes before serving.

Enjoy!

Nutritional information per serving: Kcal: 35, Protein: 2.9g, Carbs: 10.3g, Fats: 0.4g

4.   Orange Carrot Juice

Ingredients:

1 large orange, peeled

1 small carrot, sliced

1 small banana, sliced

2 whole plums, chopped

Preparation:

Peel the orange and divide into wedges. Cut each wedge in half and set aside.

Wash and peel the carrot. Cut into thin slices and set aside.

Peel the banana and cut into small chunks. Set aside.

Wash the plums and cut in half. Remove the pits and cut into bite-sized pieces. Set aside.

Now, combine orange, carrot, banana, and plums in a juicer and process until juiced. Transfer to a serving glass and add some ice before serving.

Nutritional information per serving: Kcal: 214, Protein: 4.2g, Carbs: 64.5g, Fats: 1.1g

5.   Grapefruit Beet Juice

Ingredients:

1 whole grapefruit, peeled

1 whole beet, chopped

1 small zucchini, chopped

1 cup of fresh basil, roughly chopped

1 tbsp of liquid honey

Preparation:

Peel the grapefruit and divide into wedges. Cut each wedge in half and set aside.

Wash and trim off the beet. Slightly peel and cut into bite-sized pieces. Set aside.

Peel the zucchini and chop into small chunks. Set aside.

Wash the basil thoroughly under cold running water. Slightly drain and roughly chop it. Set aside.

Now, combine grapefruit, beet, zucchini, and basil in a juicer and process until juiced. Transfer to a serving glass and stir in the honey.

Add some crushed ice before serving and enjoy!

Nutritional information per serving: Kcal: 192, Protein: 5.4g, Carbs: 38.4g, Fats: 1.1g

6.   Broccoli Kale Juice

Ingredients:

2 cups of broccoli, chopped

2 cups of kale, roughly chopped

2 medium-sized asparagus spears, trimmed

1 cup of fresh mint, torn

1 whole lemon, peeled

1 small ginger knob, peeled

Preparation:

Trim off the outer leaves of the broccoli. Wash it and cut into bite-sized pieces. Set aside.

Rinse the kale under cold running water. Slightly drain and torn with hands. Set aside.

Wash the asparagus and trim off the woody ends. Cut into small pieces and set aside.

Wash the mint and roughly chop it. You can soak it in water for 5 minutes before preparation, but it's optional. Set aside.

Peel the ginger knob and set aside.

Peel the lemon and cut lengthwise in half. Set aside.

Now, combine broccoli, kale, asparagus, ginger, mint, and lemon in a juicer. Process until juiced. Transfer to a serving glass and refrigerate for 15 minutes before serving.

Nutritional information per serving: Kcal: 118, Protein: 13.3g, Carbs: 35.3g, Fats: 2.4g

7.   Cranberry Kiwi Juice

Ingredients:

1 cup of cranberries, chopped

1 whole kiwi, peeled

1 small Granny Smith's apple, cored

1 small orange, peeled

¼ tsp of cinnamon, ground

Preparation:

Wash the cranberries and place them in a bowl. Chop into small pieces and set aside.

Peel the kiwi and cut into bite-sized pieces. Set aside.

Wash the apple and cut in half. Remove the core and cut into small pieces. Set aside.

Peel the orange and divide into wedges. Cut each wedge in half and set aside.

Now, combine cranberries, kiwi, apple, and orange in a juicer. Process until juiced.

Transfer to a serving glass and stir in the cinnamon. Add some crushed ice and serve immediately.

Nutritional information per serving: Kcal: 183, Protein: 3.1g, Carbs: 58.5g, Fats: 0.9g

8.   Watermelon Guava Juice

Ingredients:

1 cup of watermelon, chopped

1 whole guava, chunked

1 cup of pomegranate seeds

1 cup of cucumber, sliced

1 tbsp of liquid honey

Preparation:

Cut the watermelon lengthwise. For one cup, you will need a large slice. Peel and cut into small pieces. Remove the seeds and set aside. Reserve the rest for some other juices.

Peel the guava and cut into small chunks. Set aside.

Cut the top of the pomegranate fruit using a sharp paring knife. Slice down to each of the white membranes inside of the fruit. Pop the seeds into a measuring cup and set aside.

Wash the cucumber and cut into thin slices. Fill the measuring cup and reserve the rest in the refrigerator. Set aside.

Now, combine watermelon, guava, pomegranate, and cucumber in a juicer and process until juiced. Transfer to a serving glass and stir in the honey.

Add some ice and serve immediately.

Nutritional information per serving: Kcal: 134, Protein: 4.1g, Carbs: 37.5g, Fats: 1.8g

9.   Cherry Mango Juice

Ingredients:

1 cup of organic cherries, pitted

1 cup of mango, chunked

1 cup of fresh spinach, roughly chopped

1 cup of mustard greens, chopped

Preparation:

Wash the cherries and remove the stems. Cut each cherry in half and remove the pits. Fill the measuring cup and reserve the rest for later.

Peel the mango and cut into small chunks. Fill the measuring cup and reserve the rest for later.

Combine spinach and mustard greens in a large colander. Rinse thoroughly under cold water. Slightly drain and roughly chop it. Set aside.

Now, combine cherries, mango, spinach, and mustard greens in a juicer and process until juiced. Transfer to a serving glass and refrigerate for 10 minutes before serving.

Enjoy!

Nutritional information per serving: Kcal: 209, Protein: 10.6g, Carbs: 59.6g, Fats: 2.1g

10.   Zucchini Lemon Juice

Ingredients:

1 small zucchini, chopped

1 whole lemon, peeled

1 medium-sized carrot, sliced

1 cup of green grapes

1 tbsp of liquid honey

Preparation:

Wash the zucchini and cut into bite-sized pieces. Set aside.

Peel the lemon and cut lengthwise in half. Set aside.

Wash the carrot and slightly peel it. Cut into thin slices and set aside.

Wash the grapes and fill the measuring cup. Set aside.

Now, combine zucchini lemon, carrot, and grapes in a juicer and process until juiced. Transfer to a serving glass and stir in the honey.

Refrigerate for 15 minutes before serving.

Enjoy!

Nutritional information per serving: Kcal: 163, Protein: 3.2g, Carbs: 37.7g, Fats: 1.1g

11.   Artichoke Basil Juice

Ingredients:

1 medium-sized artichoke, chopped

1 cup of fresh basil, torn

1 cup of sweet potatoes, cubed

1 small green apple, cored

Preparation:

Trim off the outer leaves of the artichoke using a sharp paring knife. Wash it and cut into bite-sized pieces. Set aside.

Wash the basil thoroughly under cold running water. Sligthly drain and roughly chop it. Set aside.

Peel the sweet potatoes and cut into small cubes. Fill the measuring cup and reserve the rest for later. Set aside.

Wash the apple and cut in half. Remove the core and cut into bite-sized pieces. Set aside.

Now, combine artichoke, basil, potatoes, and apple in a juicer. Process until juiced and transfer to a serving glass.

Stir in the turmeric and serve immediately.

Nutritional information per serving: Kcal: 202, Protein: 7.6g, Carbs: 60.4g, Fats: 0.7g

12.   Pepper Broccoli Juice

Ingredients:

1 large red bell pepper, chopped

1 cup of broccoli, chopped

1 cup of Brussels sprouts, halved

1 cup of Romaine lettuce, shredded

1 cup of Swiss chard, torn

Preparation:

Wash the bell pepper and cut in half. Remove the seeds and chop into small pieces. Set aside.

Wash the broccoli and trim off the outer leaves. Cut into bite-sized pieces and fill the measuring cup. Reserve the rest for later. Set aside.

Wash the Brussels sprouts and trim off the outer wilted layers. Cut each in half and set aside.

Combine lettuce and Swiss chard in a colander. Rinse thoroughly under cold running water. Torn with hands and set aside.

Now, combine bell pepper, broccoli, Brussels sprouts, lettuce, and Swiss chard in a juicer and process until juiced. Transfer to a serving glass and refrigerate for about 10-15 minutes before serving.

You can stir in some turmeric for some extra taste. However, it's optional.

Nutritional information per serving: Kcal: 92, Protein: 8.4g, Carbs: 26.7g, Fats: 1.3g

13.   Cauliflower Avocado Juice

Ingredients:

5 cauliflower flowerets, chopped

1 cup of avocado, cubed

1 whole lime, peeled

1 whole leek, chopped

Preparation:

Wash the cauliflower flowerets thoroughly and chop into small pieces. Set aside.

Peel the avocado and cut in half. Remove the pit and cut into small cubes. Fill the measuring cup and reserve the rest in the refrigerator. Set aside.

Peel the lime and cut lengthwise in half. Set aside.

Wash the leek and cut into small pieces. Set aside.

Now, combine cauliflower, avocado, lime, and leek in a juicer and process until juiced. Transfer to a serving glass and refrigerate for 10 minutes before serving.

Enjoy!

Nutritional information per serving: Kcal: 268, Protein: 5.7g, Carbs: 32.4g, Fats: 22.5g

14.   Kale Cucumber Juice

Ingredients:

2 cups of fresh kale, chopped

1 cup of cucumber, sliced

1 medium-sized green bell pepper, chopped

1 cup of watercress, torn

1 cup of fresh parsley, torn

1 oz of water

Preparation:

Wash the kale thoroughly under cold running water. Chop into small pieces and set aside.

Wash the cucumber and cut into thin slices. Fill the measuring cup and reserve the rest for later. Set aside.

Wash the bell pepper and cut in half. Remove the seeds and chop into small pieces. Set aside.

Combine watercress and parsley in a colander. Rinse well under cold running water and torn with hands. Set aside.

Now, combine kale, cucumber, bell pepper, watercress, and parsley in a juicer and process until juiced. Transfer to a serving glass and stir in the water. Add some ice before serving.

Enjoy!

Nutritional information per serving: Kcal: 86, Protein: 9.6g, Carbs: 23.4g, Fats: 2g

15. Strawberry Lemon Juice

Ingredients:

10 large strawberries, chopped

1 whole lemon, peeled

1 cup of raspberries

1 small green apple, cored

¼ tsp of cinnamon, ground

Preparation:

Wash the strawberries and remove the stems. Cut into small pieces and set aside.

Peel the lemon and cut lengthwise in half. Set aside.

Wash the raspberries using a colander. Rinse under cold water and slightly drain. Set aside.

Wash the apple and cut in half. Remove the core and cut into bite-sized pieces. Set aside.

Now, combine strawberries, lemon, raspberries, and apple in a juicer and process until juiced. Transfer to a serving glass and stir in the cinnamon.

Add some ice and serve immediately.

Nutritional information per serving: Kcal: 151, Protein: 3.9g, Carbs: 53.5g, Fats: 3.9g

16.   Blackberry Beet Juice

Ingredients:

1 cup of fresh blackberries

1 cup of beets, trimmed

1 whole lime, peeled

1 medium-sized orange, peeled

Preparation:

Wash the blackberries thoroughly under cold running water. Slightly drain and set aside.

Wash the beets and trim off the green parts. Slightly peel and cut into thin slices. Fill the measuring cup and reserve the rest for later. You can keep the greens for some other juice.

Peel the lime and cut lengthwise in half. Set aside.

Peel the orange and divide into wedges. Cut each wedge in half and set aside.

Now, combine blackberries, beets, lime, and orange in a juicer and process until juiced. Transfer to a serving glass and add some crushed ice.

Enjoy!

Nutritional information per serving: Kcal: 135, Protein: 5.6g, Carbs: 45.9g, Fats: 1.1g

17.   Squash Cabbage Juice

Ingredients:

1 cup of butternut squash, chopped

1 cup of purple cabbage, chopped

1 large carrot, sliced

1 cup of fresh basil leaves, torn

1 oz of water

Preparation:

Peel the squash and cut in half. Scoop out the seeds and cut one large wedge. Cut into bite-sized pieces and fill the measuring cup. Wrap the rest in a plastic foil and store in the refrigerator for later.

Wash the cabbage and chop into small pieces. Fill the measuring cup and set aside.

Wash and peel the carrot. Cut into thin slices and set aside.

Rinse the basil leaves under cold running water. Roughly chop it and set aside.

Now, combine squash, cabbage, carrot, and basil in a juicer and process until juiced. Transfer to a serving glass and stir in the water. You can add a pinch of salt or red pepper if you like, but it's optional.

Serve immediately.

Nutritional information per serving: Kcal: 98, Protein: 4.1g, Carbs: 30.5g, Fats: 0.6g

18.   Tomato Parsley Juice

Ingredients:

1 cup of cherry tomatoes, halved

1 cup of fresh parsley, chopped

1 cup of cucumber, sliced

1 large red bell pepper, chopped

1 slice of onion

¼ tsp of salt

Preparation:

Wash the cherry tomatoes and remove the stems. Cut each tomato in half and set aside.

Wash the parsley thoroughly and torn with hands. Set aside.

Wash the cucumber and cut into thin slices. Fill the measuring cup and reserve the rest for later. Set aside.

Wash the bell pepper and cut in half. Remove the seeds and cut into small pieces. Set aside.

Soak onion slice in salted water for 5 minutes to reduce the bitterness.

Now, combine tomatoes, parsley, cucumber, bell pepper, and onion in a juicer and process until juiced. Transfer to a serving glass and stir in the salt.

Enjoy!

Nutritional information per serving: Kcal: 73, Protein: 4.6g, Carbs: 20.2g, Fats: 1.2g

19.   Apricot Cherry Juice

Ingredients:

2 whole apricots, pitted

1 cup of cherries, pitted

1 whole lemon, peeled

1 cup of fresh mint, chopped

1 small red apple, cored

Preparation:

Wash the apricots and cut in half. Remove the pits and chop into bite-sized pieces. Set aside.

Wash the cherries using a colander. Cut each cherry in half and remove the pits and set aside.

Peel the lemon and cut lengthwise in half. Set aside.

Wash the mint thoroughly and slightly drain. Roughly chop it and set aside.

Wash the apple and cut in half. Remove the core and cut into small pieces. Set aside.

Now, combine apricots, cherries, lemon, mint, and apple in a juicer and process until well juiced. Transfer to a serving glass and add few ice cubes before serving.

Enjoy!

Nutritional information per serving: Kcal: 195, Protein: 4.5g, Carbs: 59.1g, Fats: 1.1g

20.   Sweet Potato Apple Juice

Ingredients:

1 cup of sweet potatoes, cubed

1 small Granny Smith's apple, cored

1 cup of beet greens, chopped

1 cup of mustard greens, chopped

1 large yellow bell pepper, chopped

Preparation:

Peel the sweet potato and cut into small cubes. Fill the measuring cup and reserve the rest for later.

Wash the apple and cut in half. Remove the core and cut into bite-sized pieces. Set aside.

Combine beet greens and mustard greens in a colander. Wash under cold running water and slightly drain. Roughly chop it and set aside.

Wash the bell pepper and cut in half. Remove the seeds and cut into small pieces. Set aside.

Now, combine potatoes, apple, beet greens, mustard greens, and pepper in a juicer and process until juiced. Transfer to a serving glass and serve immediately.

You can add a pinch of salt, but it's optional.

Nutritional information per serving: Kcal: 219, Protein: 7.1g, Carbs: 62.4g, Fats: 1.1g

21.   Blueberry Guava Juice

Ingredients:

1 cup of blueberries

1 whole guava, chopped

1 large orange, peeled

1 cup of fresh mint, torn

1 small ginger knob

1 oz of coconut water

Preparation:

Wash the blueberries thoroughly using a colander. Set aside.

Peel the guava and chop into small pieces. Set aside.

Peel the orange and divide into wedges. Cut each wedge in half and set aside.

Wash the mint thoroughly and slightly drain. Set aside.

Now, combine blueberries, guava, orange, mint, and ginger in a juicer and process until well juiced. Transfer to a serving glass and stir in the coconut water.

Enjoy!

Nutritional information per serving: Kcal: 178, Protein: 5.3g, Carbs: 55.7g, Fats: 1.5g

22.　Avocado Mango Juice

Ingredients:

1 cup of avocado, cubed

1 cup of mango, chopped

1 medium-sized carrot, sliced

1 cup of cucumber, sliced

1 whole lime, peeled

Preparation:

Peel the avocado and cut in half. Remove the pit and cut into bite-sized pieces. Fill the measuring cup and reserve the rest for later. Set aside.

Peel the mango and cut into small chunks. Fill the measuring cup and reserve the rest in the refrigerator. Set aside.

Wash and peel the carrot. Cut into thin slices and set aside.

Wash the cucumber and cut into thin slices. Fill the measuring cup and reserve the rest for later.

Peel the lime and cut lengthwise in half. Set aside.

Now, combine avocado, mango, carrot, cucumber, and lime in a juicer and process until well juiced.

Transfer to a serving glass and serve immediately.

Nutritional information per serving: Kcal: 324, Protein: 5.4g, Carbs: 48.9g, Fats: 22.8g

23.   Pineapple Celery Juice

Ingredients:

1 cup of pineapple, chunked

1 large celery stalk, chopped

1 whole kiwi, peeled

1 small peach, chopped

1 oz of coconut water

Preparation:

Cut the top of a pineapple and peel it using a sharp knife. Cut into small chunks and fill the measuring cup. Reserve the rest of the pineapple in a refrigerator.

Wash the celery and cut into bite-sized pieces. Set aside.

Peel the kiwi and cut lengthwise in half. Set aside.

Wash the peach and cut in half. Remove the pit and cut into small pieces. Set aside.

Now, combine pineapple, celery, kiwi, and peach in a juicer and process until well juiced. Transfer to a serving glass and stir in the coconut water.

Add some crushed ice and serve immediately.

Nutritional information per serving: Kcal: 156, Protein: 3.3g, Carbs: 46.1g, Fats: 0.9g

24.   Apple Cinnamon Juice

Ingredients:

1 medium-sized Granny Smith's apple, cored

¼ tsp of cinnamon, ground

1 cup of cucumber, sliced

1 cup of fresh mint, chopped

1 oz of water

Preparation:

Wash the apple and cut lengthwise in half. Remove the core and cut into bite-sized pieces. Set aside.

Wash the cucumber and cut into thin slices. Fill the measuring cup and reserve the rest for later. Set aside.

Wash the mint thoroughly under cold running water. Slightly drain and chop it. Set aside.

Now, combine apple, cucumber, mint, and cinnamon in a juicer. Process until well juiced. Transfer to a serving glass and stir in the water.

Add some ice and serve.

Nutritional information per serving: Kcal: 95, Protein: 2.1g, Carbs: 28.4g, Fats: 0.6g

25.   Mango Cantaloupe Juice

Ingredients:

1 cup of mango, chunked

1 medium-sized wedge of cantaloupe

2 whole cherries, pitted

2 medium-sized strawberries, chopped

1 oz of coconut water

Preparation:

Peel the mango and cut into small chunks. Fill the measuring cup and reserve the rest in the refrigerator. Set aside.

Cut the cantaloupe in half. Scoop out the seeds and cut the wedge. Peel it and cut into chunks. Reserve the rest of the cantaloupe in a refrigerator.

Wash the cherries and cut in half. Remove the pits and set aside.

Wash the strawberries and remove the stems. Cut into bite-sized pieces and set aside.

Now, combine mango, cantaloupe, cherries, and strawberries in a juicer and process until well juiced. Transfer to a serving glass and stir in the coconut water.

Add few ice cubes and serve immediately.

Nutritional information per serving: Kcal: 124, Protein: 2.3g, Carbs: 34.8g, Fats: 0.8g

26. Lemon Grapefruit Juice

Ingredients:

1 whole lemon, peeled

1 whole grapefruit, wedged

1 medium-sized blood orange, peeled

1 medium-sized banana, chunked

¼ tsp of ginger, ground

Preparation:

Peel the lemon and cut lengthwise in half. Set aside.

Peel the grapefruit and orange. Divide into wedges and cut each wedge in half. Set aside.

Peel the banana and cut into chunks. Set aside.

Now, combine lemon, grapefruit, orange, and banana in a juicer. Process until well juiced. Transfer to a serving glass and stir in the ginger.

Refrigerate for 10 minutes before serving.

Nutritional information per serving: Kcal: 241, Protein: 5.1g, Carbs: 73.9g, Fats: 1.1g

27.   Pepper Celery Juice

Ingredients:

1 large red bell pepper, chopped

1 medium-sized celery stalk, chopped

1 cup of green peas

1 cup of fresh spinach, torn

¼ tsp of salt

¼ tsp of red pepper, ground

Preparation:

Wash the bell pepper and cut lengthwise in half. Remove the seeds and chop into small pieces. Set aside.

Wash the celery stalk and cut into small pieces. Set aside.

Rinse the green peas using a colander. Place them in a bowl and soak in water for at least 30 minutes before using. You can also cook peas to soften. However, it's optional.

Wash the spinach thoroughly and slightly drain. Torn with hands and set aside.

Now, combine bell pepper, celery, peas, and spinach in a juicer and process until juiced. Transfer to a serving glass and stir in the salt and pepper.

Serve immediately.

Nutritional information per serving: Kcal: 160, Protein: 16.9g, Carbs: 40.8g, Fats: 2.1g

28.   Basil Lime Juice

Ingredients:

2 cups of fresh basil, chopped

1 whole lime, peeled

1 cup of mustard greens, chopped

1 cup of beet greens, chopped

1 whole cucumber, sliced

Preparation:

Combine basil, mustard greens, and beet greens in a large colander. Wash thoroughly under cold running water. Roughly chop it and soak in lukewarm water for 10 minutes.

Peel the lime and cut lengthwise in half. Set aside.

wash the cucumber and cut into thin slices. Set aside.

Now, combine basil, lime, mustard greens, beet greens, and cucumber in a juicer and process until well juiced. Transfer to a serving glass and refrigerate for 20 minutes before serving.

Enjoy!

Nutritional information per serving: Kcal: 67, Protein: 6.1g, Carbs: 20.1g, Fats: 0.9g

29.   Collard Greens Avocado Juice

Ingredients:

2 cups of collard greens, torn

1 cup of avocado, cubed

1 cup of beets, chopped

1 cup of watercress, torn

¼ tsp of balsamic vinegar

¼ tsp of salt

Preparation:

Wash the collard greens thoroughly under cold running water. Place them in a bowl and add 2 cups of boiling water. Let it soak for 10 minutes. slightly drain and set aside.

Peel the avocado and cut in half. Remove the pit and cut into small cubes. Fill the measuring cup and reserve the rest in the refrigerator. Set aside.

Wash the beets and trim off the green ends. Peel and cut into small pieces. Set aside.

Wash the watercress and torn with hands. Set aside.

Now, combine collard greens, avocado, beets, and watercress in a juicer. Process until well juiced and transfer to a serving glass. Stir in the vinegar and salt for some extra taste.

Refrigerate for 10 minutes before serving.

Nutritional information per serving: Kcal: 258, Protein: 8.2g, Carbs: 30.2g, Fats: 22.7g

30.   Asparagus Lemon Juice

Ingredients:

2 cups of asparagus, chopped

1 whole lemon, peeled

1 cup of cucumber, sliced

1 cup of fresh parsley, torn

Preparation:

Wash the asparagus and trim off the woody ends. Cut into small pieces and set aside.

Peel the lemon and cut lengthwise in half. Set aside.

Wash the cucumber and cut into thin slices. Fill the measuring cup and reserve the rest for later.

Wash the parsley thoroughly under cold running water and slightly drain. Torn with hands and set aside.

Now, combine asparagus, lemon, cucumber, and parsley in a juicer and process until well juiced. Transfer to a serving glass and refrigerate for 15 minutes before serving.

Enjoy!

Nutritional information per serving: Kcal: 64, Protein: 8,6g, Carbs: 21.5g, Fats: 1.1g

31.　Vanilla Blackberry Juice

Ingredients:

1 cup of blackberries

¼ tsp of vanilla extract

1 cup of pomegranate seeds

5 large strawberries, chopped

1 large banana, peeled

Preparation:

Place the blackberries in a colander and rinse under cold water. Slightly shake to drain and set aside.

Cut the top of the pomegranate fruit using a sharp paring knife. Slice down to each of the white membranes inside of the fruit. Pop the seeds into a measuring cup and set aside.

Wash the strawberries and remove the stems. Cut into small pieces and set aside.

Peel the banana and cut into small chunks. Set aside.

Now, combine blackberries, pomegranate, strawberries, banana, and vanilla extract in a juicer and process until juiced.

Transfer to a serving glass and add some crushed ice.

Serve immediately.

Nutritional information per serving: Kcal: 249, Protein: 7.5g, Carbs: 81.9g, Fats: 3.2g

32.   Avocado Mint Juice

Ingredients:

1 cup of avocado, chunked

1 cup of fresh mint, chopped

2 whole kiwis, peeled

3 whole plums, chopped

1 oz of water

Preparation:

Peel the avocado and cut lengthwise in half. Remove the pit and cut into small chunks. Fill the measuring cup and reserve the rest in the refrigerator. Set aside.

Wash the mint thoroughly under cold running water. Roughly chop it and set aside.

Peel the kiwis and cut lengthwise in half. Set aside.

Wash the plums and cut in half. Remove the pits and cut into bite-sized pieces. Set aside.

Now, combine avocado, mint, kiwis, and plums in a juicer and process until juiced. Transfer to a serving glass and stir in the water.

Refrigerate for 10 minutes before serving.

Enjoy!

Nutritional information per serving: Kcal: 356, Protein: 6.9g, Carbs: 59.4g, Fats: 23.5g

33. Spinach Fennel Juice

Ingredients:

1 cup of fresh spinach, torn

1 cup of fennel, sliced

1 medium-sized celery stalk, chopped

1 medium-sized artichoke, chopped

Preparation:

Wash the spinach thoroughly under cold running water. Slightly drain and torn with hands. Set aside.

Wash the fennel bulb and trim off the wilted outer layers. Cut into small pieces and fill the measuring cup. Reserve the rest for some other juice.

Wash the celery stalk and cut into bite-sized pieces. Set aside.

Trim off the outer leaves of the artichoke using a sharp paring knife. Wash it and cut into bite-sized pieces. Set aside.

Now, combine spinach, fennel, celery, and artichoke in a juicer and process until well juiced. Transfer to a serving glass and refrigerate for 10 minutes before serving. You can add some salt to taste, but it's optional.

Nutritional information per serving: Kcal: 80, Protein: 11.5g, Carbs: 28.6g, Fats: 1.3g

34.   Papaya Mango Juice

Ingredients:

1 cup of papaya, chunked

1 cup of mango, chopped

1 whole apricot, chopped

1 small ginger knob, peeled

2 oz of coconut water

Preparation:

Peel the papaya and cut into small chunks. Fill the measuring cup and reserve the rest in the refrigerator. Set aside.

Peel the mango and cut into small pieces. Fill the measuring cup and reserve the rest for later. Set aside.

Wash the apricot and cut in half. Remove the pit and cut into bite-sized pieces. Set aside.

Peel the ginger knob and set aside.

Now, combine papaya, mango, apricot, and ginger in a juicer and process until juiced. Transfer to a serving glass and stir in the coconut water.

Add some crushed ice and enjoy!

Nutritional information per serving: Kcal: 160, Protein: 1.2g, Carbs: 45.3g, Fats: 1.2g

35.   Pineapple Orange Juice

Ingredients:

1 cup of pineapple chunks

1 small orange, peeled

1 cup of blackberries

1 small peach, pitted

¼ tsp of vanilla extract

Preparation:

Cut the top of a pineapple and peel it using a sharp paring knife. Cut into small chunks and fill the measuring cup. Reserve the rest of the pineapple in a refrigerator.

Peel the orange and divide into wedges. Set aside.

Place the blackberries in a colander and rinse thoroughly under cold running water. Set aside.

Wash the peach and cut in half. Remove the pit and cut into small pieces. Set aside.

Now, combine pineapple, orange blackberries, and peach in a juicer and process until juiced.

Transfer to a serving glasses and stir in the vanilla extract. Add few ice cubes and serve immediately.

Nutritional information per serving: Kcal: 184, Protein: 5g, Carbs: 59.2g, Fats: 1.3g

36. Carrot Zucchini Juice

Ingredients:

1 large carrot, sliced

1 small zucchini, chopped

1 small green apple, cored

1 whole lemon, peeled

¼ tsp of ginger, ground

Preparation:

Wash and peel the carrot. Cut into thin slices and set aside.

Peel the zucchini and cut into thin slices. set aside.

Wash the apple and cut in half. Remove the core and cut into bite-sized pieces. Set aside.

Peel the lemon and cut lengthwise in half. Set aside.

Now, combine carrot, zucchini, apple, and lemon in a juicer. Process until well juiced. Transfer to a serving glass and stir in the ginger.

Add some ice and serve.

Nutritional information per serving: Kcal: 116, Protein: 3.4g, Carbs: 35.6g, Fats: 0.9g

37.   Mango Basil Juice

Ingredients:

1 whole mango, chunked

1 cup of basil, torn

4 medium-sized strawberries, chopped

1 whole kiwi, peeled

Preparation:

Peel the mango and cut into small chunks. Set aside.

Rinse the basil thoroughly under cold running water and slightly drain. Torn with hands and set aside.

Wash the strawberries and remove the stems. Cut into bite-sized pieces and set aside.

Peel the kiwi and cut lengthwise in half. Set aside.

Now, combine mango, basil, strawberries, and kiwi in a juicer and process until juiced. Transfer to a serving glass and add some ice before serving.

Enjoy!

Nutritional information per serving: Kcal: 230, Protein: 4.6g, Carbs: 64.7g, Fats: 1.9g

38. Apple Green Tea Juice

Ingredients:

1 medium-sized Granny Smith's apple, cored

1 cup of fresh mint, torn

1 whole lemon, peeled

1 medium-sized celery stalk

1 tsp of green tea

1 tbsp of liquid honey

Preparation:

Wash the apple and cut in half. Remove the core and cut into bite-sized pieces. Set aside.

Wash the mint thoroughly under cold running water. Torn with hands and set aside.

Peel the lemon and cut lengthwise in half. Chop into quarters and set aside.

Place green tea in a small bowl. Add two tablespoons of hot water and let it soak for 5 minutes.

Wash the celery stalk and chop it into bite-sized pieces. Set aside.

Now, combine apple, mint, lemon, celery, and green tea mixture in a juicer and process until well juiced. Transfer to a serving glass and stir in the honey.

Refrigerate for 20 minutes before serving.

Nutritional information per serving: Kcal: 163, Protein: 2.6g, Carbs: 43.1g, Fats: 0.8g

39. Cranberry Orange Juice

Ingredients:

1 cup of cranberries

1 large orange, peeled

1 whole kiwi, peeled

2 whole plums, pitted

¼ tsp of cinnamon, ground

Preparation:

Place the cranberries in a colander. Wash thoroughly under cold water and slightly drain. Set aside.

Peel the orange and divide into wedges. Cut each wedge in half and set aside.

Peel the kiwi and cut lengthwise in half. Set aside.

Wash the plums and cut each in half. Remove the pits and cut into bite-sized pieces. Set aside.

Now, combine cranberries, orange, kiwi, and plums in a juicer and process until juiced. Transfer to a serving glass and stir in the cinnamon.

Add some ice and serve immediately.

Nutritional information per serving: Kcal: 182, Protein: 3.8g, Carbs: 59.1g, Fats: 1.1g

40.   Pepper Kale Juice

Ingredients:

1 medium-sized red bell pepper, chopped

1 cup of fresh kale, torn

1 cup of fresh spinach, torn

1 large radish, sliced

1 cup of cucumber, sliced

1 oz of water

Preparation:

Wash the bell pepper and cut lengthwise in half. Remove the seeds and cut into small pieces. Set aside.

Combine kale and spinach in a colander. Wash thoroughly under cold running water and slightly drain. Torn with hands and set aside.

Wash the radish and trim off the green parts. Cut into thin slices and set aside.

Wash the cucumber and cut into thin slices. Fill the measuring cup and reserve the rest for later.

Now, combine bell pepper, kale, spinach, radish, and cucumber in a juicer and process until juiced.

Transfer to a serving glass and stir in the water. Refrigerate for 10 minutes before serving.

Enjoy!

Nutritional information per serving: Kcal: 86, Protein: 10.5g, Carbs: 22.8g, Fats: 1.9g

41.   Peach Pineapple Juice

Ingredients:

1 medium-sized peach, chopped

1 cup of pineapple, chunked

1 small zucchini, cut into bite-sized pieces

¼ tsp of ginger, ground

2 tbsp of coconut water

Preparation:

Wash the peach and cut in half. Remove the pit and cut into bite-sized pieces. Set aside.

Using a sharp paring knife, cut the top of the pineapple. Gently remove all hard skin and slice it into thin slices. Fill the measuring cup and reserve the rest for later.

Wash the zucchini and cut into bite-sized pieces. Set aside.

Now, combine peach, pineapple, and zucchini in a juicer and process until well juiced. Transfer to a serving glass and stir in the ginger and coconut water.

Refrigerate for 10 minutes before serving.

Enjoy!

Nutritional information per serving: Kcal: 141, Protein: 3.7g, Carbs: 41.6g, Fats: 0.9g

42.   Mango Strawberry Juice

Ingredients:

1 cup of mango, chunked

½ cup of strawberries, cut into bite-sized pieces

1 small apple, cored

2 whole cherries, pitted

1 tsp of dried mint, ground

Preparation:

Peel the mango and cut into bite-sized pieces. Set aside.

Wash the strawberries and remove the core. Cut into bite-sized pieces and set aside.

Wash the apple and cut in half. Remove the core and cut into small pieces. Set aside.

Wash the cherries and cut each in half. Remove the pits and set aside.

Place the mint in a small bowl and add two tablespoons of hot water. Let it soak for 5 minutes.

Now, combine mango, strawberries, apple, cherries and mint mixture in a juicer and process until juiced. Transfer to a serving glass and refrigerate for 15 minutes before serving.

Enjoy!

Nutritional information per serving: Kcal: 185, Protein: 2.8g, Carbs: 53.8g, Fats: 1.1g

43.   Pomegranate Beet Juice

Ingredients:

2 cups of pomegranate seeds

1 cup of beets, sliced

1 cup of watercress, chopped

1 cup of fresh basil, chopped

¼ tsp of ginger, ground

Preparation:

For two cups of pomegranate seeds, you'll need about two medium-sized pomegranate fruits. First, cut the top of each pomegranate fruit using a sharp paring knife. Slice down to each of the white membranes inside of the fruit. Pop the seeds into a measuring cups and set aside.

Wash the beets and trim off green ends. Chop into bite-sized pieces and fill the measuring cup. Reserve the rest for later.

Combine watercress and basil in a colander. Rinse thoroughly under cold running water. Drain and roughly chop it. Set aside.

Now, combine pomegranate seeds, beets, watercress, and basil in a juicer and process until well juiced. Transfer to a serving glass and stir in the ginger.

Refrigerate for 10 minutes before serving.

Enjoy!

Nutritional information per serving: Kcal: 166, Protein: 6.6g, Carbs: 46.6g, Fats: 2.5g

44.   Melon Parsnip Juice

Ingredients:

1 large wedge of honeydew melon

1 cup of parsnips, sliced

1 medium-sized carrot, sliced

1 cup of cucumber, sliced

¼ tsp of ginger, ground

Preparation:

Cut one large honeydew melon wedge and peel it. Remove the seeds and cut into bite-sized pieces. Wrap the rest of the melon in a plastic foil and refrigerate.

Wash and slightly peel the parsnips. Cut into thin slices and fill the measuring cup. Reserve the rest for later. Set aside.

Wash and peel the carrot. Cut into thin slices and set aside.

Wash the cucumber and cut into slices. Fill the measuring cup and reserve the rest for later.

Now, combine melon, parsnips, carrot, and cucumber in a juicer and process until juiced. Transfer to a serving glass and stir in the ginger. Refrigerate for 10 minutes before serving.

Enjoy!

Nutritional information per serving: Kcal: 152, Protein: 3.4g, Carbs: 46.2g, Fats: 0.9g

ADDITIONAL TITLES FROM THIS AUTHOR

70 Effective Meal Recipes to Prevent and Solve Being Overweight: Burn Fat Fast by Using Proper Dieting and Smart Nutrition

By Joe Correa CSN

48 Acne Solving Meal Recipes: The Fast and Natural Path to Fixing Your Acne Problems in Less Than 10 Days!

By Joe Correa CSN

41 Alzheimer's Preventing Meal Recipes: Reduce or Eliminate Your Alzheimer's Condition in 30 Days or Less!

By Joe Correa CSN

70 Effective Breast Cancer Meal Recipes: Prevent and Fight Breast Cancer with Smart Nutrition and Powerful Foods

By Joe Correa CSN